Essentials of Sleep

For Fitness

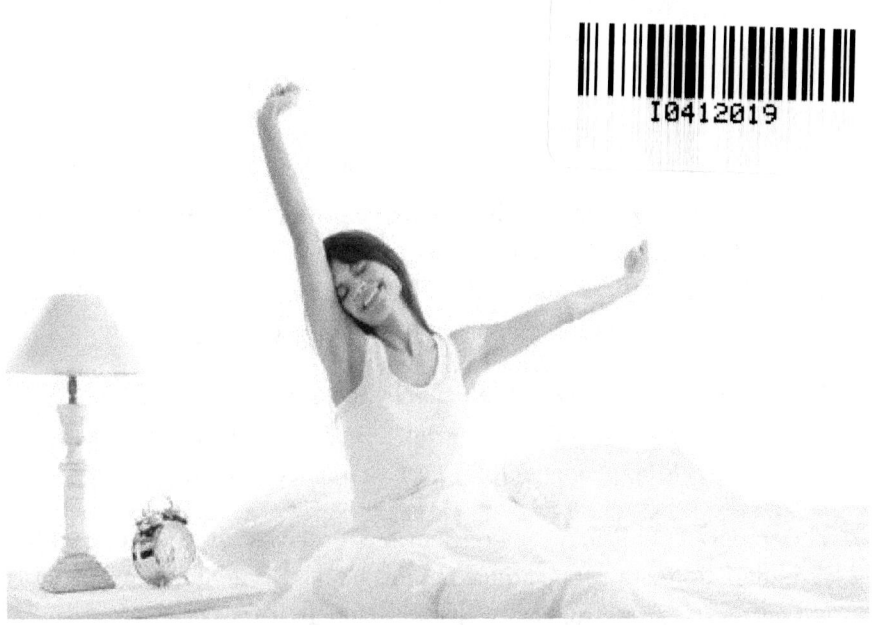

Health Learning Series

M. Usman

Mendon Cottage Books

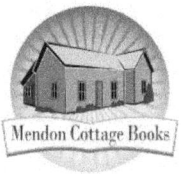

JD-Biz Publishing

Our books are available at

1. Amazon.com
2. Barnes and Noble
3. Itunes
4. Kobo
5. Smashwords
6. Google Play Books

Table of Contents

Prelude

Sleep is probably the most underrated entity in the fast paced environment of the 21st century. More and more people are trying to increase their working hours as their work load increases, while keeping their leisure time unchanged; this can only come from shortening their sleeping time. Even though at first this might sound like a win-win situation, it's actually not. The sleep quality and quantity are linearly dependent on each other, so one can't stay up while the other's down.

Sleep hygiene is a term which can effectively describe the quality of one's sleep. It is basically a combination of different practices which must be topped up in order to get a normal sleep during night time and a proper level of awareness during the day. It is an important component of one's health and experts believe that it's not something to be left to the mind; one should actively participate in building time for his/her sleep which requires conscious discipline. Sleep hygiene is not only responsible for correcting a person's cognitive abilities but can also improve a person's physical functions. It is one of the first steps when it comes to treating people with sleeping disorders like disruptions and apnea. As you read the book, you will find that improving a person's sleep can effectively protect him against asthma, thyroid disease, and heart failure.

In short, one can dramatically improve his/her lifestyle by giving proper attention to his sleep. This book will tell you the impact of proper sleep on the body and how a person can improve the standard of his/her sleep.

Getting Started

Chapter # 1: Optimal Sleep

Sleep is a dynamic quantity; at some point in life people need a lesser amount of sleep than they did when they were younger. It is constantly affected by our ever changing lifestyle and health. A new born, for instance, has an average sleeping time of 16 hours, while a teenager, on the other hand, sleeps 9 hours a day. Adults sleep less than 9 hours, but try to keep their sleeping time above 6 hours. Women in their pregnancy months bear the pressure of a whole other human being and thus, to process all the vitals for the baby, need more sleep. Being pregnant is not the only parameter that judges the need to sleep more; sleep also depends on the level of tiredness and quantity of sleep one is getting. If a person accumulates too little sleeping time in the previous days, he/she has to compensate for that by sleeping extra time in the coming days; otherwise the person will suffer from not only, low mood and error in judgment, but also with impaired bodily functions.

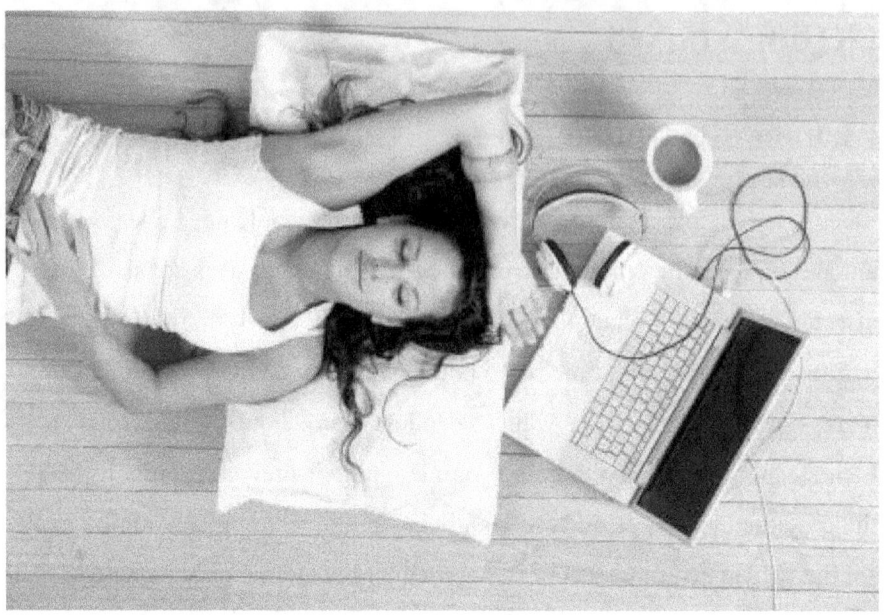

Some people treat these errors by taking a short nap, but in the long run this sleeplessness is not cured and only a short boost in alertness is produced. Napping is inefficient and thus, only a portion of benefits of a night's sleep are obtained, which means that it is not the cure. Another way in which people tend to fulfill their sleep requirements is by sleeping more on the weekends or their days off. This abnormality indicates that more time needs to be allocated to sleep during normal days. Moreover, sleeping more on specific days while sleeping less on others would only play with the body's internal clock and disturb it. Most people sleep only lightly and for much shorter lengths as they age, but in fact, they need almost the same amount of sleep as they did in adulthood. A study has shown that 50% of people over 65 have issues similar to insomnia which come from either aging or as side effects.

Experts believe that feeling sleepy or drowsy during work hours indicates that the body is unsatisfied with its sleeping hygiene. Moreover, experts agree that falling asleep within 5 minutes of lying down shows that a person is deprived of essential sleep. Internment episodes of sleep also indicate a lack of sleep. A table that shows normal amounts of sleep for people has been shown below:

Age	Recommended amount of Sleep
New born	16 – 18 hours a day
Pre-school	11 – 12 hours a day
School	10 hours a day
Teenage	10 hours a day
Adulthood	7 – 8 hours a day

Chapter # 2: Why is Sleep Important?

Sleeping improves cognitive, as well as physical body functions. The statement is blindly approved by many, but the exact science about this lucid state still remains mystery. Yet, there are a few things that every researcher agrees on; these are listed below:

- The core, i.e. the cells and tissues of the body, require time to repair themselves. Sleep provides the body's cells with adequate time to rejuvenate, which cannot be wholly achieved while the body is still awake. Sleeping increases the concentration of the body's hormones which are optimal for swift repair.

- Sleep disorders are becoming way too common. People are becoming more and more lethargic, losing their strength more often, and losing clarity in life. All this happens because they are deprived of their sleep which ensures a correct buildup of body's resources, meaning a steady stream of vitamins and nutrients reaching the brain as well as other organs. A deprivation of just 1.5 hours of sleep can result in a 32% decrease in mental capability, a study has shown.

- Sleep is also very important to keep a healthy sex life. Sleep deprivation can result in a loss of sexual energy, erectile dysfunction and reduced fertility. A research conducted at the University of Colorado showed that sleep deprived male individuals had almost half the amount of testosterone compared to subjects who had no sleep problems.

- Proper sleep strengthens memory, while lack of sleep leads to memory loss. An associate professor at New York University Medical Center found out that even though practice plays a big hand in making a person learn something, sleep also plays a vital part. When a person sleeps, something happens that helps the person learn and effectively memorize it. Sleep causes memory consolidation which turns short-term memories into long ones. Alzheimer's disease, which is quite an infamous disease known for its brain damage, is a direct outcome of sleep deprivation.

- Weight gain is another abnormality which is linked with improper sleep hygiene. It is one of the biggest issues of the century and is an ever increasing problem. One study in particular, has found that individuals getting less than 6 hours of sleep on a daily basis are much more prone to gaining weight than those getting adequate sleep. The study also reported that people who slept at least 8 hours a night had the lowest percentage of body fat. No researcher has been able to accurately report the reasons to it, but a theory that floats around, links the amount of sleep to the amount of hormones in the body which cause weight management. Obstructed sleep results in higher levels of a hormone called ghrelin and lower levels of leptin, while also showing decreased levels of insulin which disturb the whole natural order of the body; all these factors then contribute to weight gain. Thus, in order to neutralize another factor that leads to weight loss, sleep another hour in the bed instead of putting one in the gym.

- The Immunity system is also affected by the amount of sleep a person gets. Losing sleep increases many inflammatory compounds in the body like CRPs, interleukins, etc. which damage cells in the body. Research at Rush University showed that sleep deprivation in a chronic manner can lead to inflammatory diseases, which can in turn chronic.

- People getting sleep of less than 7 hours each night are at a much greater risk of developing cardiovascular disorders and diabetes, than those who sleep their designated amount of time. Studies have shown that people sleeping less than 6 hours develop type II diabetes at a higher rate, while another study showed that decreased sleeping hours lead to cardiovascular diseases. This is directly attributed to the increase in stress hormone levels.

- That is not all; sleep has also been found to decrease life expectancy! A research that targeted chronically sleep deprived individuals getting less than 6 hours a day, showed that sleep deprivation caused as much damage to life as smoking or heart disease. Another study confirmed this finding and stated a relative risk of 1.12 which meant a very close association between dying and having insomnia.

These were some of the cons of sleeping less; hopefully they will wake you up and put you on the path to a better sleep, which is explained ahead.

Chapter # 3: Purpose of Sleep

At this stage, there won't be any doubt as to why sleep is essential and a vital part of daily life. Still, many people have the habit to question a lot of things around them, even the purpose of their existence. So, the question regarding the purpose of sleep won't come as a surprise. Forget a normal individual, even scientists some time get confused on the dynamics of sleep; despite all the countless hours of research, scholars are still not sure as to why a person sleeps and the purpose of it.

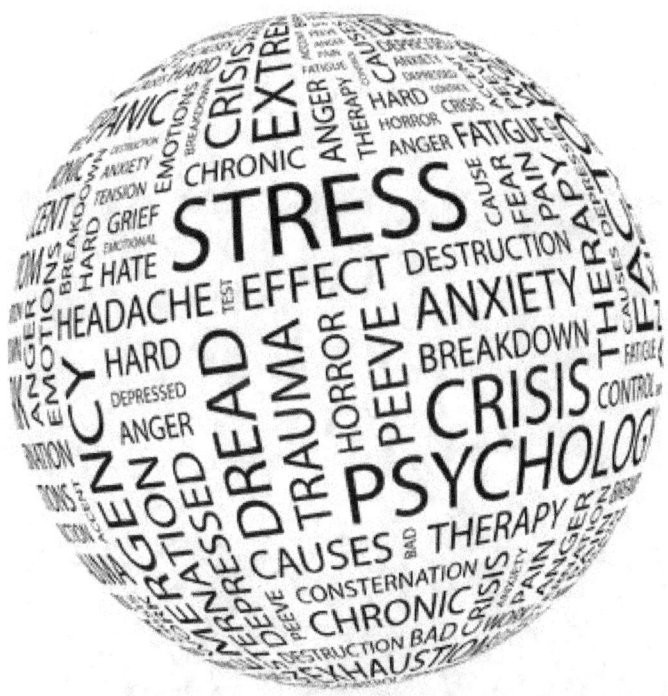

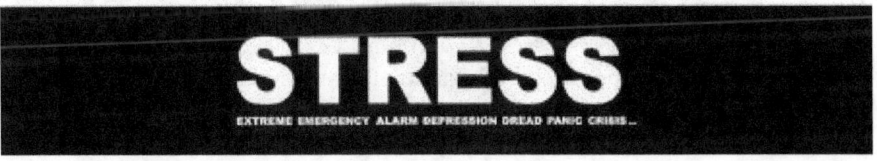

But, it doesn't end here; several theories have been developed regarding the purpose of sleep and several continue to float as no scientist has been able to prove a single theory true or false. Most of these theories are in one way or another related to evolution, but as stated earlier none of the theories neither stand out nor complement each other. The following are a few theories regarding sleeping, that scientists have launched:

1.   Energy conservation theory:

According to this theory, the main function of sleep is described as one that reduces a person's energy demands during that portion of the day when the search for food is at its minimum. Supporting studies that help this theory indicate that the human body's metabolism is significantly reduced during sleep.

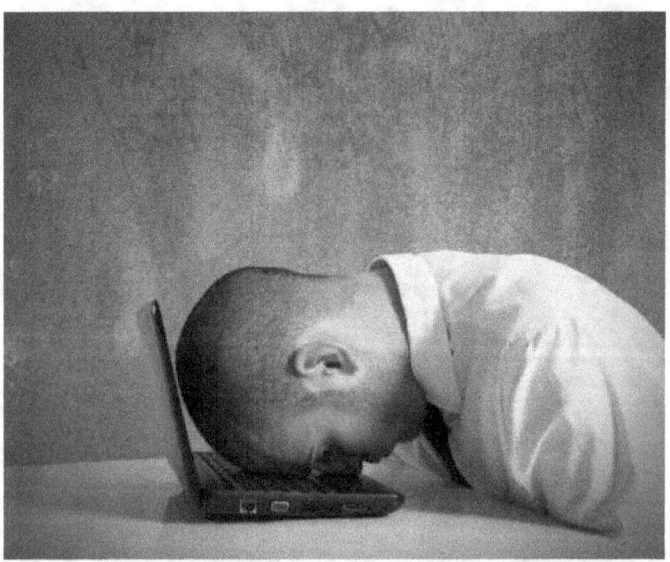

The theory is also supported by the fact that brain is just 2 percent of the body weight, but during day time it consumes almost 20 percent of the body's energy. Of course, this figure is just related to staying awake, as processing takes even more power. It must also be stated that during sleeping, the temperature of the body falls by an average of 1 degree Celsius, which means a decrease in energy expenditures. This may sound like a palpable theory, but if the numbers are looked at in greater detail, the energy expenditures break down. The 10 percent reduction in energy is equal to the energy obtained from banana or an apple. Another aspect that must be considered at the same time is that during REM sleep, the metabolic rate goes back to normal or sometimes even higher and this particular type of sleep takes 5 cycles to complete. So this theory isn't as accurate as it sounds.

2.   Restorative theory:

Another very digestible solution to the purpose of sleep is the restorative theory, which states that sleep is a state in which the body aims to restore all that is lost during the time a person is awake. Sleep provides ample time for the body to fully repair itself and if this time is not given, the body starts to suffer from many disorders and conditions.

The theory is getting more and more support after recent studies are obtaining results that are positive for the theory. A recent study at the University of Rochester has found that the brain undergoes a cleansing process during the time it sleeps. The researcher coined the term glympatic system; it is known that all the organs in the body are supplied blood through a network of blood vessels. In addition to this system of blood transfers, another network is also contained within the body known as the lymphatic system. This system is responsible for draining fluid outside the cells and injecting it back into the central circulatory system, which cleanses and rids the body of all the waste. The brain however, is deprived of the lymphatic system which means that the metabolism waste only accumulates in the body. This is where the glymphatic system comes in; during the time we are awake, the cerebrospinal fluid found in our spinal cord and brain remains static, but during sleep it starts to flow. The flow comes not only from the pool surrounding the brain, but also in between the neurons which clears up all the debris and waste that comes from metabolism. Chronic sleep deprivation means that the waste does not get cleared up which results in diseases, most notably, Alzheimer's.

3.   Brain plasticity theory:

Another very interesting theory put forward by researchers is the brain plasticity theory, which states that sleep plays an important role in developing and enhancing the function of the brain, irrespective of age. A study at the Simon Fraser University discovered that when a person is young, his/her neurons grow at top speed, but as he/she ages the growth becomes stagnant. The speed reaches its lowest levels during adulthood and starts to take a negative route as a person ages. Researchers were able to find that improving sleep hygiene resulted in an improvement in the growth of neurons. The growth was really swift in hippocampus, which is a brain area that is linked with basic cognitive behavior. It was also found that more than 24 hours of sleep deprivation had an extremely adverse effect on the hippocampus and with that, all the cognitive functions.

These were pretty much the boldest theories that try to explain the reason why people sleep, but when comes down to it, no one is able to explain this lucid behavior and why it happens. Still, decades' worth of research is needed to truly explain the need behind sleep.

Sleep Hacking

Chapter # 1: What is it?

There are many ways in which a person can ensure themselves of quality sleep. One of these methods is sleep hacking, which involves the person formulating a strategy for a better sleep. Sleep hacking improves the quality and not the quantity of sleep hours. Studies have shown that this statement is not far from the truth. Sleep hacking is becoming increasingly popular with more individuals as their work load increases. Did you know that more than 22 million people in the USA work in shifts? This means that their sleep timings get disturbed way too much, so sleep hacking comes in handy here and ensures quality sleep. Studies have shown that shift workers are at the greatest risk when it comes to getting sleep disorders, thus, sleep hacking methodology is most beneficial to these workers.

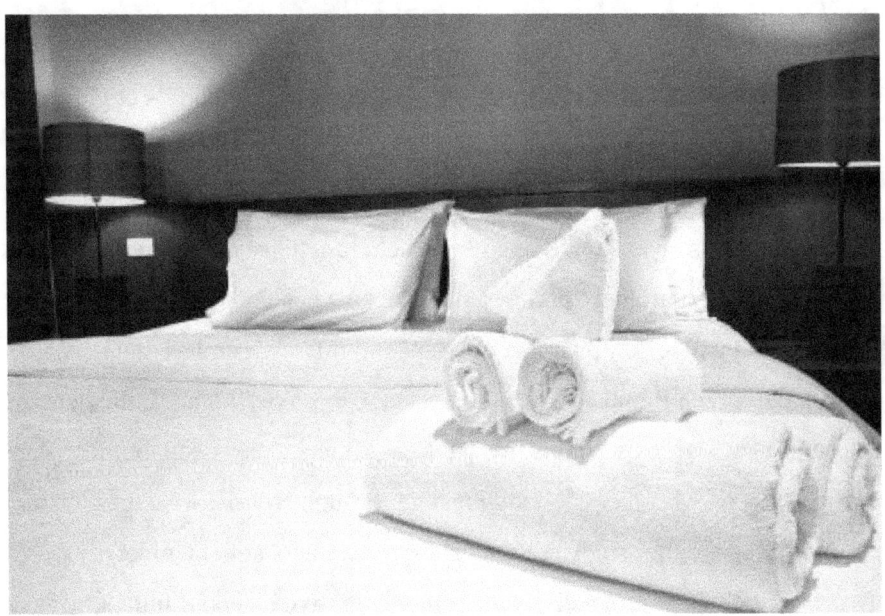

That's not all; in recent years studies have found that sleep hacking is also advantageous to medical issues that are related to fatigue, stress, etc. These issues should not be taken lightly and some of these can soon turn into serious problems like diabetes, cardiovascular conditions, and even cancers. Evidence has shown that there is a relationship between cancer and fatigue and an appropriate amount of sleep can fill this void, which ultimately leads to a lower risk of cancer. A very interesting research study made the finding that the human mind can start functioning even after getting just 2 hours of sleep. If that's right, then why do we need to spend $1/3^{rd}$ of our time in beds, when it can be utilized elsewhere? This is explained by polyphasic sleep cycles. To understand these sleep cycles, it must first be known that the sleep consists of five stages which may broadly be divided into 2 major types:

i.   Non-rapid eye movement sleep or NREM

ii.   Rapid eye movement sleep or REM

Non-REM sleep consists of four sub-stages, in which the body's cognitive as well as physical activity starts to decrease and hits a virtual stop when it reaches the 4th stage. The real dynamo starts after this stage ends and the REM one begins. The cognitive and physical functions start to increase and keep increasing until they hit the same level as when a person is awake. Research has actively shown that toddlers and infants spend as much as 7 hours a day in the Rapid Eye Movement stage. As a person ages, this length falls to 2 hours which explains the claim of 2 hours a day sleep, but in order to reach this REM stage, the body must go through Non-REM stages, which require time. Another study conducted by researchers at the University of Texas showed that brain activity and other cognitive essential functions gain their peak when the mind enters Rapid Eye Movement Stage. There is a way in which the brain can be made to quit all the other parts of sleep and skip right to the polyphasic part, which means that the body will feel replenished in just 2 hours. How do you accomplish this? Read on and you'll find out.

Chapter # 2: Ways to Optimize Sleep

The following are a number of techniques that can be employed to optimize your sleep:

1.   **Transform your bed into a recharge station**:

Get rid of all the unnecessary junk and clutter that rests in your bed more that you do. These may include books, laptops, fancy cushions, recharging wires, etc. Get rid of them and make your bed a comfort zone where you can unwind after a tiring day of work. A younger individual may feel comfortable even without a mattress, but a person above 40 is recommended to sleep on a mattress that is comfortable for his/her back.

2.   **Change your sheets:**

If you wish to minimize your lying around time and maximize your recovery time when you go to bed, choose a set of earthing sheets. These sheets may be plugged into the grounding outlet in almost every home socket; it not only helps a person relax but also help him/her sleep better.

3.   **Reduce lighting in the room:**

In order to obtain the best quality sleep, it is optimum to make your room as dark as possible. This can be achieved very easily by turning off all electric appliances that have any kind of lights or LEDS connected to them. You might not be able to see anything after this, but you will definitely have a good night's rest.

Scientists also obtained another very interesting finding on circadian rhythms. While previously researchers believed that circadian rhythm was affected by social interactions, new research shows that this statement is inaccurate. Researchers at the Max Planck Institute performed a number of experiments in which subjects were kept in sound proof rooms to eliminate every type of foreign interferences to the circadian rhythms. After that, the light intensity in that room was tweaked and the researchers discovered that light was the major factor that controlled the circadian rhythm. Light has influence over hormones like melatonin, which results in higher induction of sleep. Therefore, darker rooms cause the greatest release of melatonin and thus ensure a good night's sleep.

4. **Eliminate blue light:**

As some of you might know already, bright light consists of 7 colors, which means there are a range of wavelengths that are emitted from a laminating source. Out of all these wavelengths, blue light has the greatest frequency and red light has the least. You might also have heard from someone that using a laptop before going to bed may cause you damage or disturbances in sleep. The reasoning behind this enigma is that these appliances emit blue light in huge amounts, which cause a decrease in melatonin secretion. If you remember, melatonin is the hormone which induces comfortable sleep. But, this light interferes with the hormone and exposure to it can decrease the secretion down to just 39%.

Thus, the first choice a person has is to turn off all electrical appliances and create a completely dark environment or he/she can eliminate all sources of blue light. These need to be turned off at least an hour before going to bed as the melatonin secretion starts early. There is even another way to block out the blue light, which can be done by using special amber goggles. According to a research, these lenses have the ability to block blue light which ensures better quality sleep and sleep hygiene in general.

5.   **Turn down the thermostat:**

Sleep onset is very much related to a person's body temperature. It is believed to be a vital parameter when considering sleep. The researchers at Cornell University in New York have tried to study this relation in various ways and have succeeded in some. They found that a person's body temperature may not have any effect on a person's sleep hygiene, but it does affect the onset of sleep. So, if you wish to sleep early turn down the air conditioner a few notches.

6.   **Exercise:**

Exercise comes in everywhere, doesn't it? Well, it's been found that people who exercise tend to have healthier sleep hygiene. A daily walk not only keeps a person's mass in check, but also reduces the chances of waking up at night. Aerobic exercise in particular can boost the body's metabolism for melatonin, which induces sleep. A study reported that menopausal women, who exercised for at least 3 and a half hours a week, slept much better than those who didn't do any exercise. Still, a person should keep in his/her mind, the timing of the workout, because if a person indulges in physical activity too close to bed time, he/she can disturb his sleeping pattern, which can cause irregularities throughout the week. Thus, it is best to finish the workout at least 2 – 3 hours before bed.

This melatonin production is not the only reason exercise is recommended by professionals for a better sleep. Exercise can decrease the level of stress hormones like cortisol, which would ensure a better day time! It also increases the number of natural endorphins in the body which acts as a relaxant.

7.   **Taking a nap:**

Your body is made most sensitive by the cardiac system in between 7 AM and 9 AM, but after that it starts to drop. At 3 PM – 4 PM it reaches very low levels, which can now be used as means to sleep. The science behind this statement also revolves around melatonin. Researchers have found that the hormone keeps changing its levels throughout the day:

-    The lowest level of the serum is in between 7 and 9 in the morning.

-    The level rises between 10 and 12 in the morning.

-    It reaches its peak between 1 and 4 in the afternoon.

Furthermore, supporting evidence also indicates a decrease in the body's temperature during the latter part of the day, which suggests that the best time to nap is in between 1 and 4.

8.   **Clear your stomach:**

In this day and age, a person eats a multitude of dishes, with each one having its own distinct ingredients. Many elements in a person's meal can cause disruption in sleep like too much alcohol or sea food. The solution to this is activated charcoal, which in particular, contains elements that pick up all these toxins and cleanse the body of them. This allows the body to sleep in a better internal environment.

9.   **Keep stress in check:**

An emptied mind is very much necessary for a perfect sleep. A lot of people go to bed with their heads filed with thoughts of the whole day and this kind of mind can never let the body sleep. Even if it does, the sleep won't induce that much serenity, as having a clear mind will. Thus, try to purposefully empty your mind and reserve the sleeping time only for comfort. A very effective way to relax is to take deep breathes or engage in any other type of breathing exercise; yoga can also help you with this.

10.   **Have a pre-bed bath!**

A bath before bed time can significantly increase a person's sleep hygiene. Researchers aren't really sure about this point, but behavioral studies have shown that people, who took baths before sleeping, woke up much fresher. A possible explanation to this statement is a rise in temperature during a bath, but a drop in it soon after due to evaporation.

11.   **Essential oils:**

Having a pleasant spray or refresher in your room won't hurt you. Actually, it would do more good. Essential oils like chamomile and lavender can improve a person's sleep. A research at Wesleyan University showed that a person's sleep was improved significantly after his sleeping place was personalized with essential oils that lifted the person's mood and thus helped him sleep better.

12.   **Enter carbohydrates:**

Research has shown that a person can easily increase the chances of a good night's sleep by eating carbohydrates in a small amount. The food should be less than 200 calories, so a piece of toast or a small bowl of cereal would suffice.

The sleepy effect that comes after consumption of a carbohydrate rich diet is due to an increase in the brain's level of tryptophan. When a person consumes carbohydrates, insulin rises naturally and when insulin rises, it opens up channels for tryptophan in the brain. As much as 1g of tryptophan can increase the level of sleepiness in a person.

13. **Build a plan:**

The amount of sleep you need each day varies. Sometimes you're very tired, sometimes you've overslept the previous day, and sometimes you're just not in the mood. It's best to build a plan that will manage your sleeping times throughout the week. Firstly, choose a time when you would like to get up in the morning; now try to get up at this exact time, for 2 weeks. Don't sleep in the evening unless you're very tired. Soon, your brain will make amends and you'll be able to sleep in a scheduled manner.

14. **Polyphasic sleep:**

Now that you know the whole nine yards about sleep, it's time to move into polyphasic sleep, which would explain the benefits of sleep hacking. In general, there are 3 types of sleeps.

a.   Siesta:

This includes almost 6 hours of major sleep with 20 minutes of nap in the afternoon. This type of sleeping patter is widely found in countries located in Asia and Latin America.

b.   Everyman:

This pattern is nap friendly and involves a number of naps throughout the day. Each of the naps will take almost 60 minutes of your time so if you slept 8 hours, you are allowed to take 2 naps of 1 hour each.

c.   Uberman:

This style is for those who prefer to take only naps and no core sleep. You can have 7 – 8 naps of 20 minutes or more.

15.   **Avoid sleeping medications:**

Having a uniform and constant circadian rhythm is very vital for a person's well-being. Sleeping pills are undoubtedly the fastest way to achieve serenity, but it devastates a person's insides. Studies have shown that sleeping pills may induce sleep in the body, but in fact, they are taking away sleep from the body. They disrupt the body's circadian cycle which can result in a desynchronized body-mind balance. Using sleeping pills can also increase episodes of insomnia, so it is conclusively said that it is best to avoid sleeping pills or any other kind of medication.

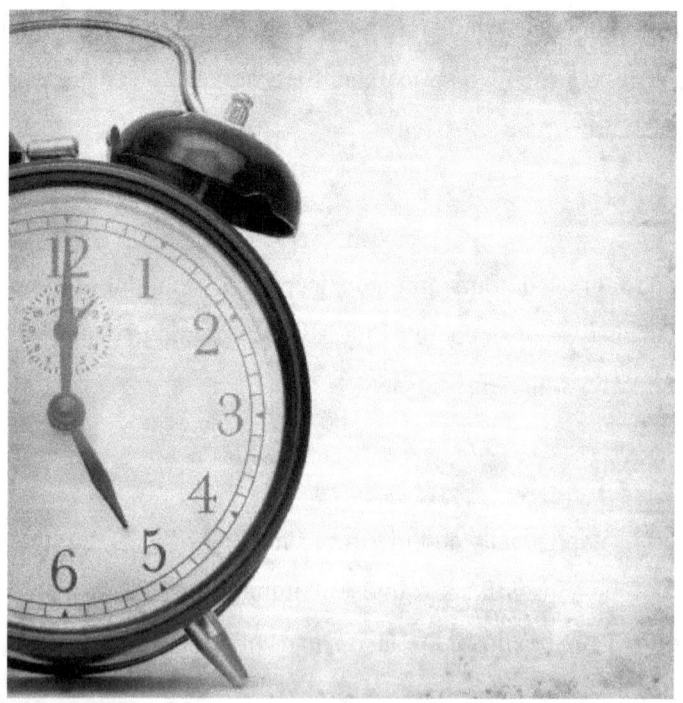

Chapter # 3: Tips to Remember

Here are a few tips you should keep in mind regarding sleep:

i.   Set regular bedtimes:

The most optimized and well-proven method to ensure better sleep hygiene is to go to bed at the same time every day and wake up at the same time. Choose any time at night and start practicing going to bed at this time. Try not to break this routine up, otherwise you'll break your rhythm, but if you ever do want to change your bed timings, just make small increments of 15 minutes every day until the desired adjustment is approached.

ii.   Wake up at the same time:

Almost everyone would like to wake up without an alarm clock. If you get up in the morning without an alarm clock, this means that you are getting enough sleep and this should be your standard time to wake up. But, as almost no one can manage to go to work late just because his/her alarm clock didn't work, try adjusting your go-to-bed time so that you need minimum assistance from the alarm clock, to get up.

iii.   Make up the lost sleep:

Sometimes you just aren't getting enough sleep, so it's a good idea to take in between naps to make up for the lost time. This will easily let you get rid of the accumulating sleep debt without alternating the internal clock. The nap should be restricted to 30 minutes and should be taken at night, because if you sleep during the day, your clock will be altered and you'll have trouble sleeping at night. The best time to nap is in between 1 PM and 4 PM as the melatonin level is highest at this time.

iv.   **Fight after-meal sleep:**

Don't go to bed after eating, as you'll most probably end up with sleep that will do you no good other than disrupting internal co-ordination between the mind and the body. Instead, try to do something that is stimulating and will keep you from falling alseep; you can either wash dishes or invite a friend over. But if you give up to the sleepiness, you'll wake up in the middle of the night.

Conclusion

Sleep is another of the countless mysteries of nature. It sounds like such a simple affair, but in reality it has far reaching effects and consequences. It's a process designed for the human body to regain its original strength after a day of hard work and it is very much essential. The people who tend to side line it, only suffer. The suffering can easily be seen in their performance, which worsens with every passing sleep-deprived night. This book is therefore designed to guide you on the right path and give required importance to sleep, as a sleep deprived person starts to fail in almost all walks of life. This is not just a shot in the dark, but actual reality. The book describes the purpose, advantages and tricks to better sleep; they are pretty much self-explanatory and any avid reader would love to go through this book. But lastly, this is just a book and you need to decide for yourself. I'm pretty sure that just like the majority, you would also prefer a satiating sleep rather than a tiring day, so follow the instructions given clearly in the book and have a good night!

Author Bio

Muhammad Usman is a distinguished medical graduate of Allama Iqbal medical college (AIMC). He is a professional writer who has been in the field for more than 4 years. During this time he has produced 10,000+ articles, blogs and eBooks on various niches related to diseases, health, fitness, nutrition and well-being. He is a regular contributor to several journals related to medicine and surgery. He is the editor of several journals and newspapers.

References

http://www.123rf.com/photo_15981293_tired-sleepy-woman-waking-up-and-yawning-with-a-stretch-while-sitting-in-bed-isolated-on-white-backg.html?term=sleep

http://www.123rf.com/photo_21907088_a-girl-laying-on-the-floor-after-surfing-on-the-internet-with-a-laptop.html?term=sleep

http://www.123rf.com/photo_17347130_concept-of-stressed-busibnessman-at-work.html?term=sleep

http://www.123rf.com/photo_9129840_stress-globe-with-different-association-terms-wordcloud-vector-illustration.html?term=sleep%20brain

http://www.123rf.com/photo_19751178_white-towels-prepared-on-bed.html?term=bed

http://www.123rf.com/photo_22480536_old-fashioned-alarm-clock.html?term=alarm

Check out some of the other JD-Biz Publishing books

Gardening Series on Amazon

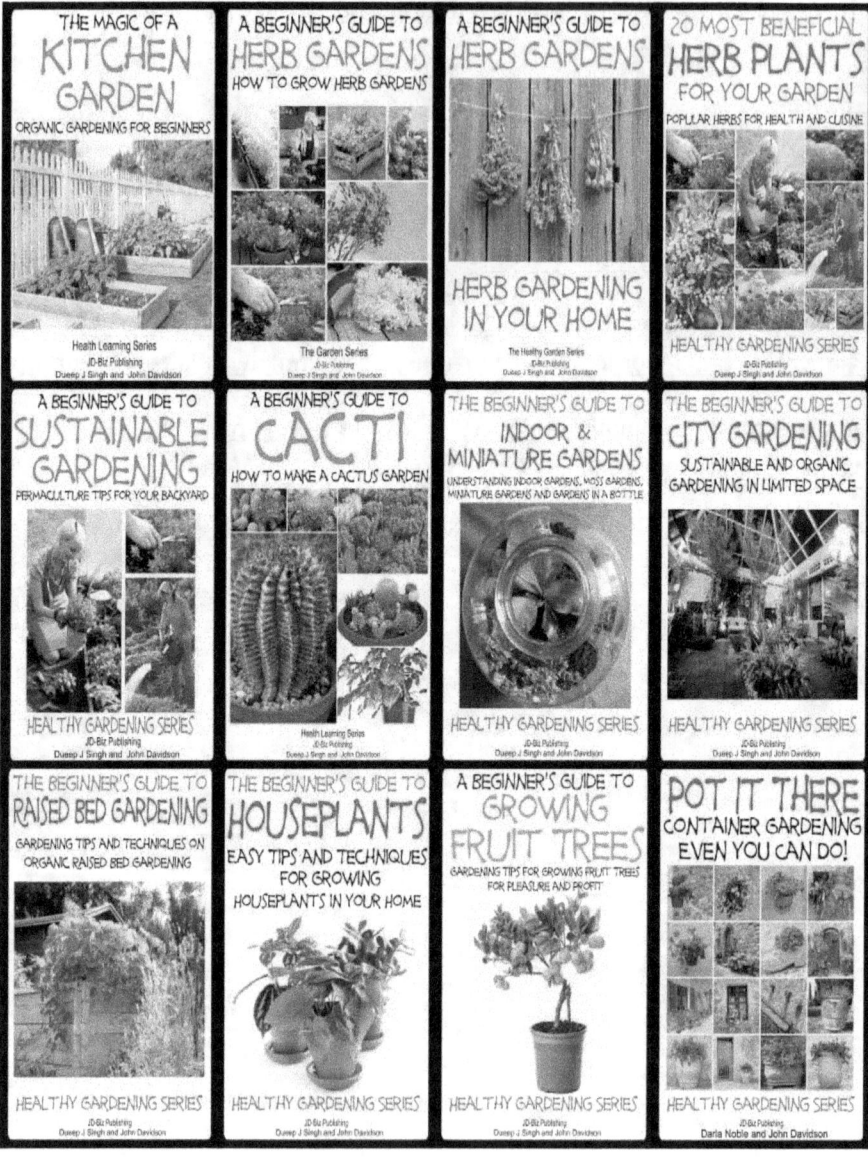

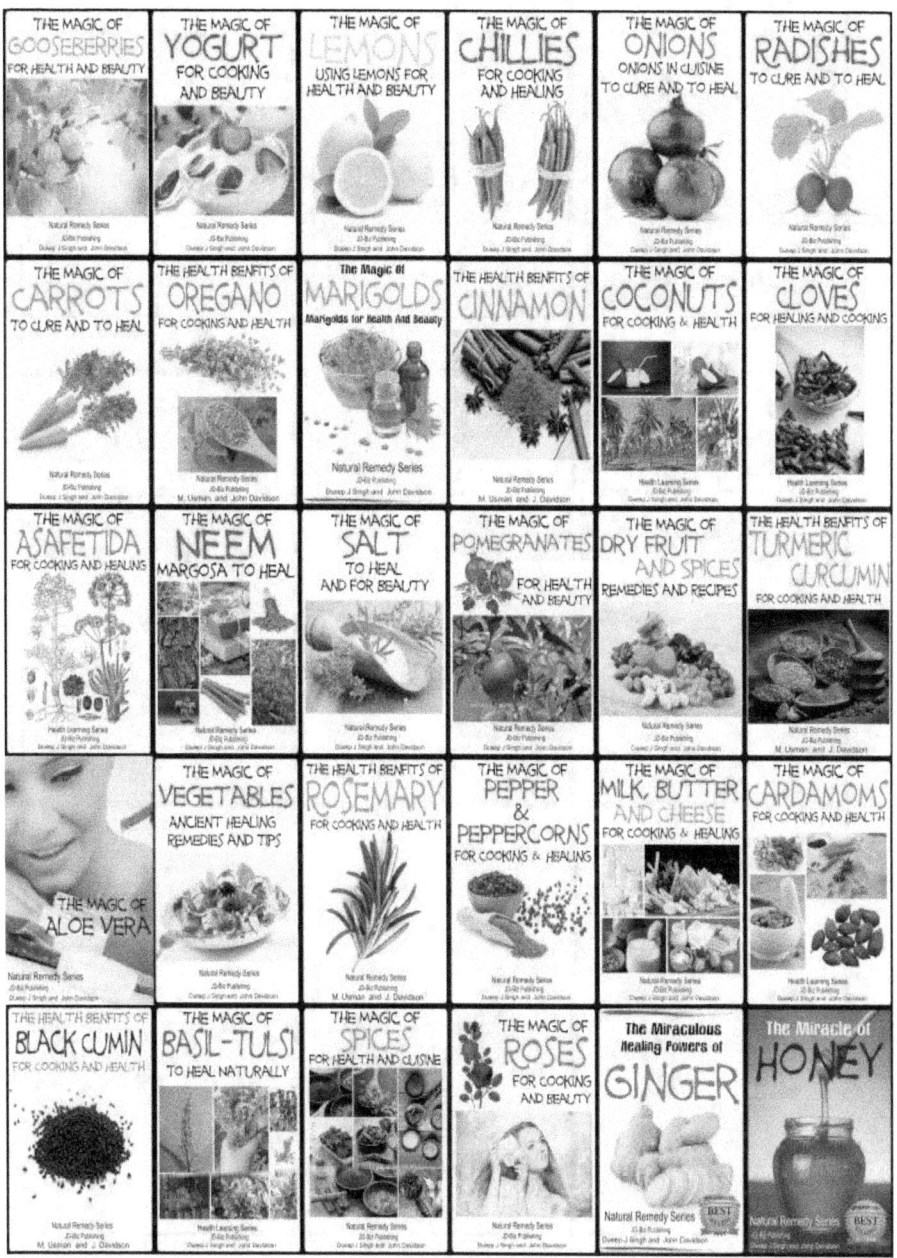

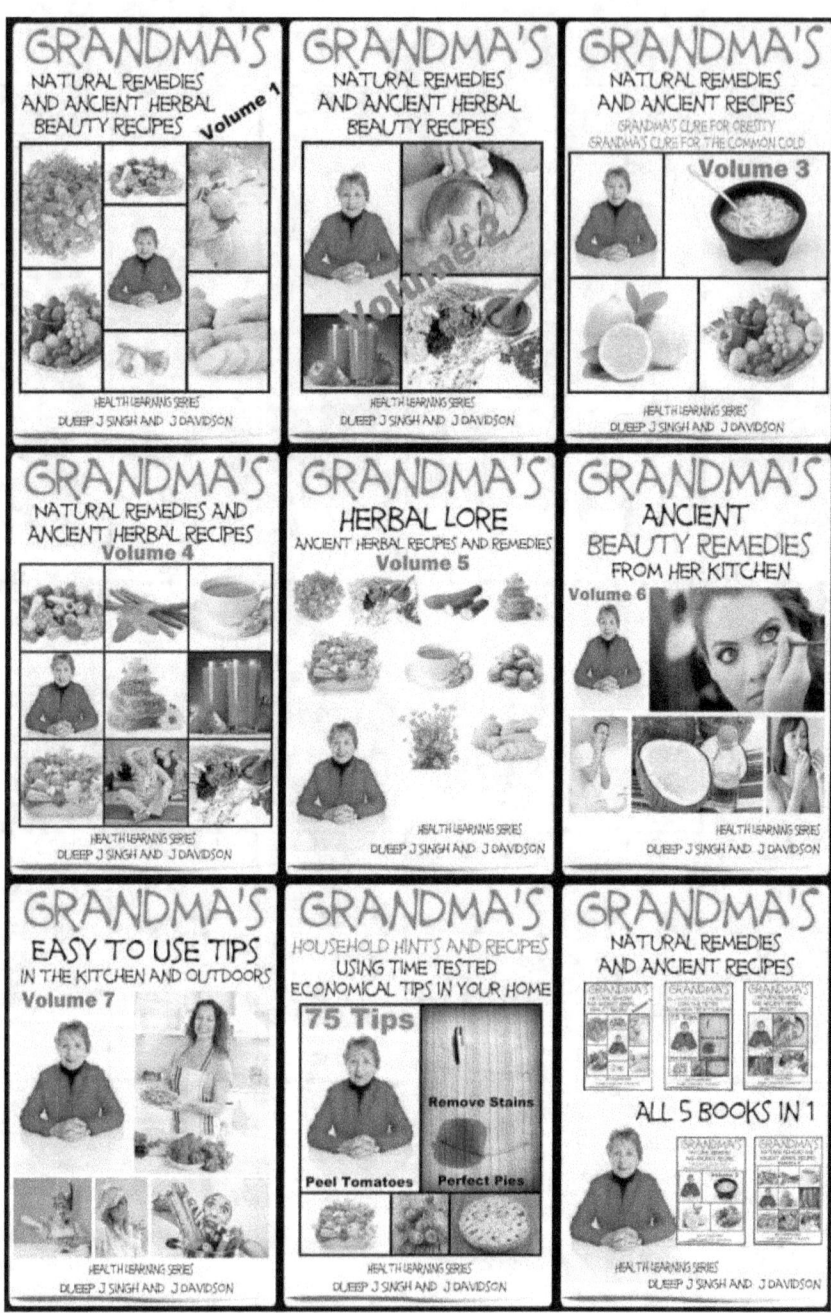

Country Life Books

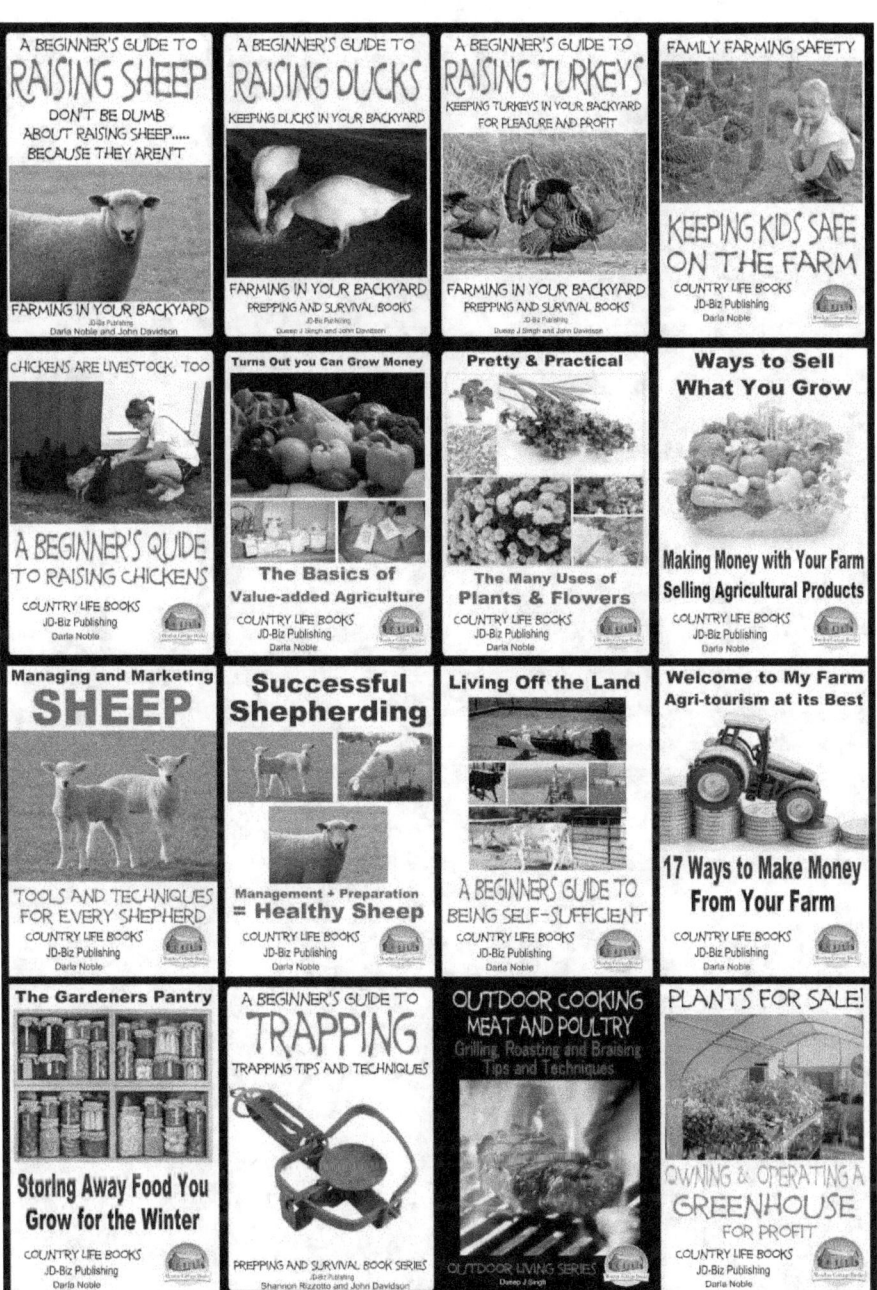

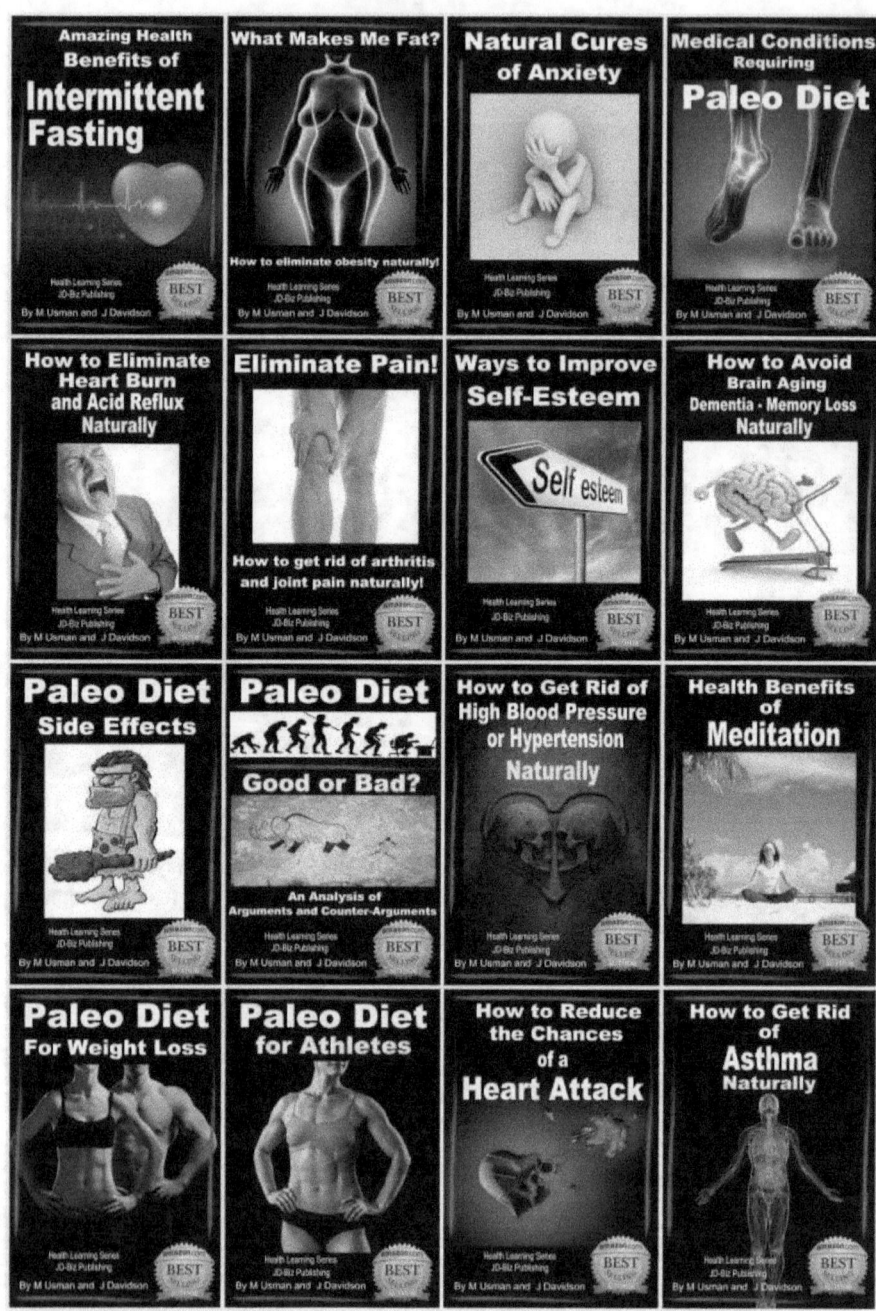

Amazing Animal Book Series

Learn To Draw Series

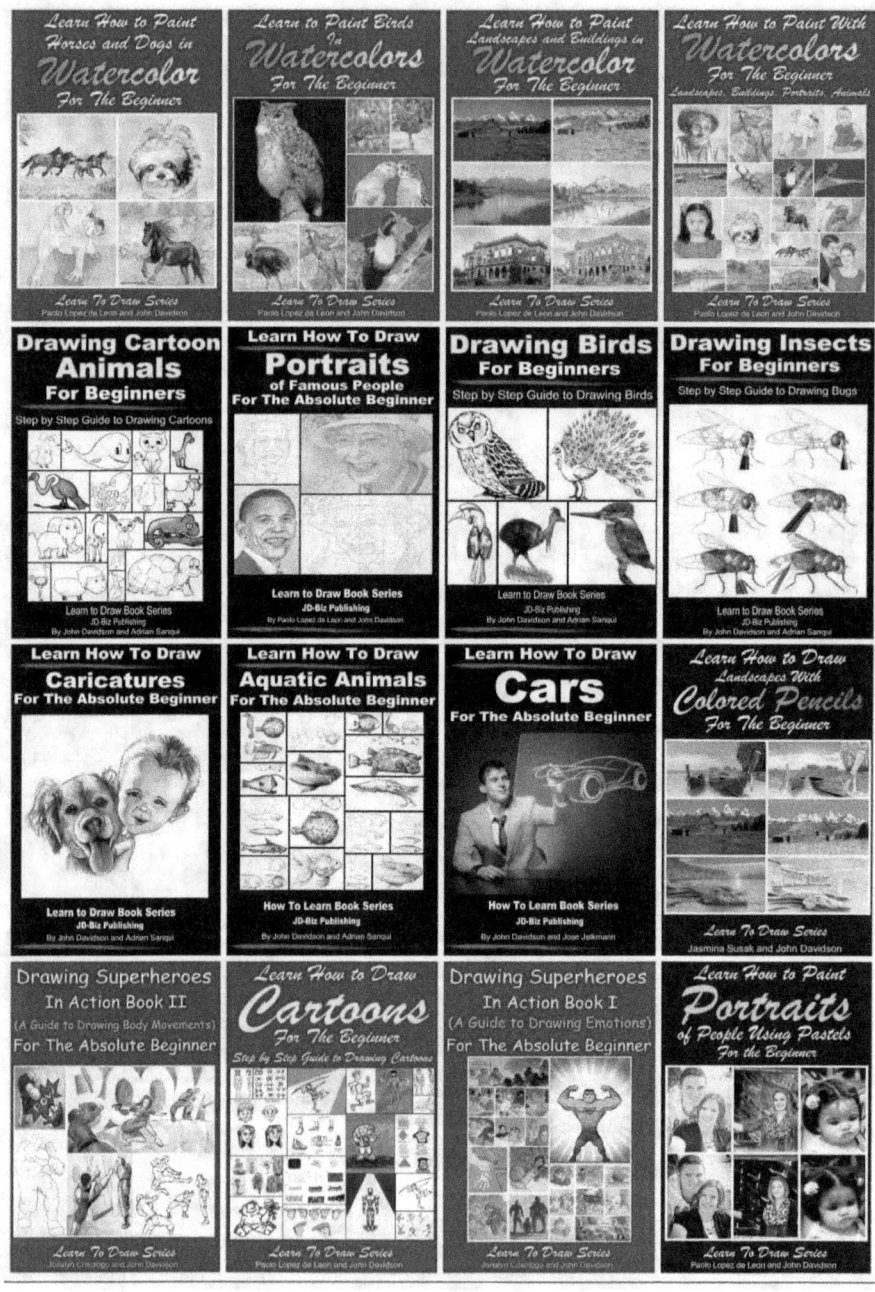

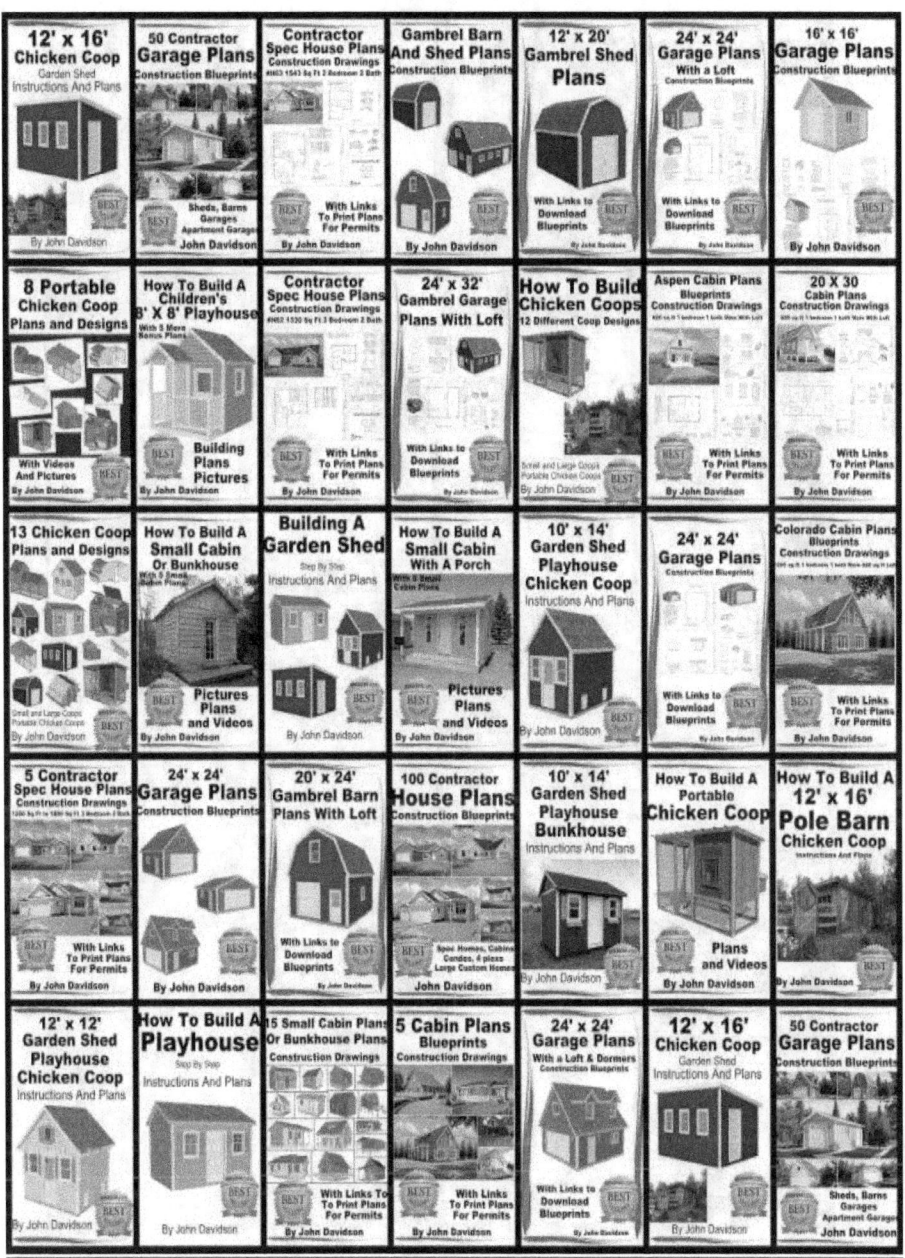

Entrepreneur Book Series

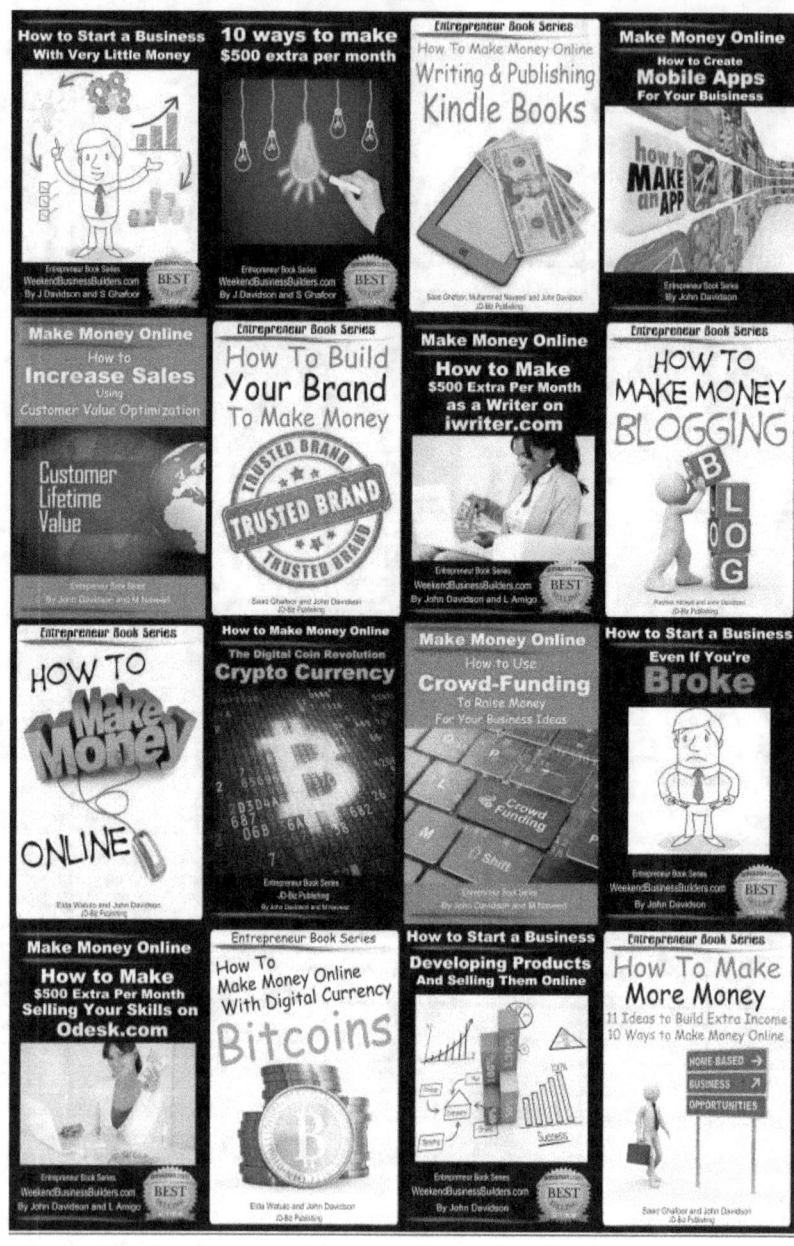

Our books are available at

1. Amazon.com

2. Barnes and Noble

3. Itunes

4. Kobo

5. Smashwords

6. Google Play Books

Publisher

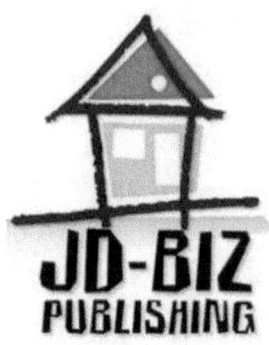

JD-Biz Corp

P O Box 374

Mendon, Utah 84325

http://www.jd-biz.com/

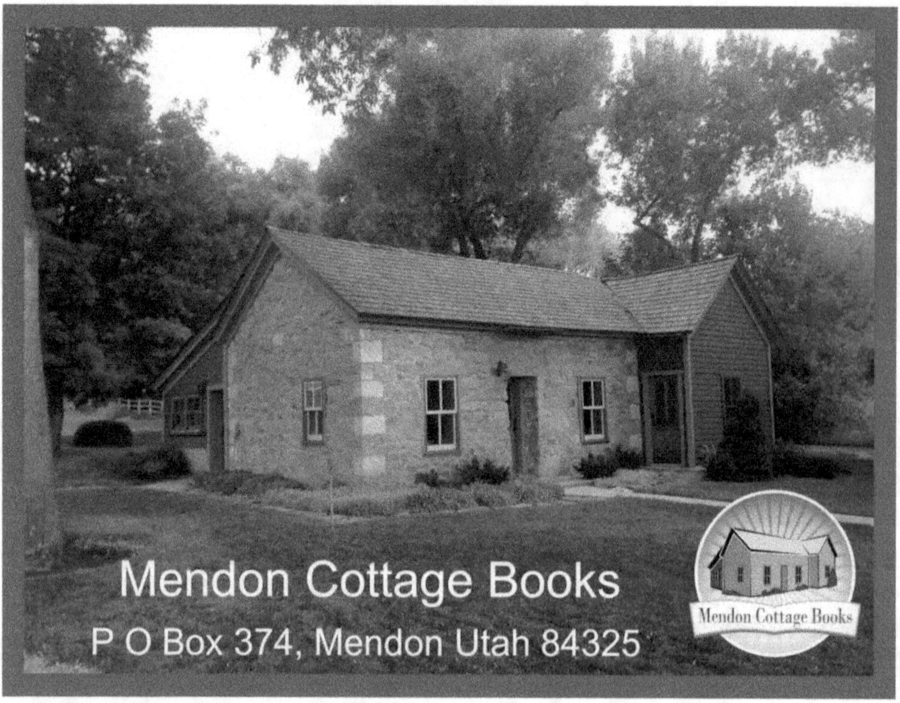

Mendon Cottage Books

P O Box 374, Mendon Utah 84325